The High Triglycerides Diet

The Ultimate Guide to Lowering your Triglycerides with a 21-Day Meal Plan

By

Anna Keating

The High Triglycerides Diet

Copyright © 2018

ISBN: 9781977036650

Warning and Disclaimer

Every effort has been made to make this book as accurate as possible. However, no warranty or fitness is implied. The information provided is on an "as-is" basis. The author and the publisher shall have no liability or responsibility to any person or entity with respect to any loss or damages that arise from the information in this book.

Publisher Contact

Skinny Bottle Publishing

books@skinnybottle.com

Introduction

High triglycerides in your blood can cause a series of health complications. From artery clogging and heart diseases to even fatal strokes in some extreme cases. No, I am not saying this to scare you but to motivate you to take control over your life.

What goes into your mouth lives a mark on your blood picture. Once you test your blood you can easily see whether you need to cut back on the fatty stuff, skip the sugar, or even boost up on some minerals. If you are reading this now, chances are you already know that the only way to lower your triglycerides is by changing your diet and lifestyle, completely.

Although triglycerides don't get as much attention as LDL cholesterol does, they can be just as harmful. Knowing what not to eat and what to consume can not only help you bring them back within the normal range, but it can also support your heart health in the long run.

Whether you want to lower your triglycerides or are simply looking for dietary advice on how to keep them balanced, this book has a lot to teach you on that subject. From how they get increased and why they matter to how to lower them through dietary changes, this guide will help you not only drop the high triglycerides, but boos your goof HDL cholesterol as well.

And if that's not enough, I've got a yummy 21-day meal plan to get you started. Stick with me and let's get rid of the unhealthy fats together.

What are Triglycerides?

Most people hear about triglycerides after they get spooked about their high levels shown on their blood test results. But unlike cholesterol and blood sugar – things that we know we should fear – most of us have no idea what the function of the triglycerides is.

When we think about the fat in our body, we usually think about the cholesterol. After all, isn't the cholesterol what we have been warned to keep a track of? Good and bad cholesterol, saturated and unsaturated fat, it seems that preventing a heart disease requires a complex system of fat tracking. Add triglycerides on top of that and you might as well give up and dive into a bowl of deep-fried food, right?

You may think it is overwhelming but understanding these fat types is simple. And triglycerides are the easiest to comprehend.

Triglyceride is the name for the main fat that is found in your body. When you think about that fat that hugs your belly or sticks to your hips after eating a carb-loaded meal, you are actually thinking about the triglycerides.

Triglycerides come from the food we eat. The more calories we consume, the more triglycerides our body will build. The main source of triglycerides are the carbohydrates. And just like carbs, the triglycerides can also be used for energy. They can be either stored in the liver or sent throughout the bloodstream to be stored intramuscularly and provide tissues with energy.

Think about it this way. When we eat our body does a calorie selection. It chooses to use some of them immediately, while the ones that it doesn't need at that moment, get converted into triglycerides. They are then stored in the fat cells, and later released by hormones, for energy. Obviously, if you eat more calories than you burn, you most likely have more triglycerides than what's considered normal.

It is the liver who is in charge of building the triglycerides from raw fatty acids and glucose elements. The name comes from their structure: the liver builds glucose into a glycerol chain, which 3 fatty acids are later attached to. When the body needs energy, it breaks down the fatty acids from the base of glycerol. Once broken, these fatty acids enter the muscles and into the mitochondria, where they produce energy. If there are excess fatty acids and not that much energy requirement, these fatty acids get back to the liver, become reattached to the glycerol chain, and create other triglyceride levels that must be stored.

Triglycerides vs Cholesterol

Because they are both types of fat and can contribute to heart disease, people often use cholesterol and triglycerides interchangeably. But even though they are both transported through the bloodstream by lipoproteins and can both lead to cardiovascular and circulatory issues, cholesterol and triglycerides represent two different things.

The main difference between these two is in the way in which they perform inside the body. Triglycerides represent the fat that gets broken by the body and gets burned to provide energy. Cholesterol, on the other hand, is used to build cells and hormones within the body. Another difference is that the body doesn't necessarily need the dietary cholesterol since it can produce it on its own. When it comes to triglycerides, however, the body relies on the food consumption to create them, since they cannot be produced otherwise.

Neither triglycerides nor cholesterol can mix with the blood. That's why the liver sends them throughout the bloodstream packaged in packages called *lipoproteins*. Lipoproteins is what transports these fats. There are three types of lipoproteins: low density lipoproteins called LDL, very low-density lipoproteins called VLDL, and high-density lipoproteins, which are called HDL. The LDL is what we refer to the *bad cholesterol*, and the HDL is *the good cholesterol*.

The triglycerides have a pretty tight relationship with the good cholesterol HDL. The triglyceride/HDL ratio can be a good indicator of how risky your fat levels are.

Detecting High Triglycerides

Triglycerides represent the most common fat type in our bodies. They are essential for energy and for the balance of our overall health. However, in excess amount, triglycerides can be extremely dangerous and cause some serious health problems.

Having high triglyceride levels is indeed a sign of concern. Unfortunately, most of the people who have excessive amounts of this type of fat are unaware of the risk that they are exposed to.

From who is at risk, how to detect them, and just how risky they are, this chapter will clear all the confusion you may have about triglycerides and help you address the problem accordingly.

Who's at Risk?

To put it simply, everyone. The more calories we consume, the more triglycerides we have in our bloodstream. And if we take into consideration this modern junk-food and low-activity modern lifestyle that most of us are used to, it is no surprise that the number of people suffering from high triglyceride and cholesterol levels has skyrocketed in the past few decades, and it seems to be only going upwards.

However, it is not only the raise in calories that increased the levels of the triglycerides. There are many risk factors that can contribute to the increase of this type of fat in the blood. Here are the most common ones:

Age. Unfortunately, it is in our human nature to be prone to having increased triglyceride levels with age. As we get older, the number of triglycerides in our bloodstream rises.

Weight. Remember how we said that the triglycerides represent the fat that is glued to our bellies hips, and thighs? Well, it is no surprise that overweight people are at risk for having high triglyceride levels. The riskiest group are those people who have a waist measure above 35 inches.

Activity Level. Sedentary lifestyle is bad for every aspect of your health, and the triglyceride levels are no exception. The less you move, the fewer calories you burn, which eventually results in gaining weight and having more fat around your waist. And since triglycerides represent our bodily fat, it is obvious how inactivity can lead to high triglyceride levels. It's a simple math, really. The more inactive you are, the higher your chance of a heart disease.

Alcohol Consumption. It has been scientifically proven that alcohol consumption raises the triglyceride levels. And if you are a regular drinker, well, chances are you have more triglycerides in your blood than you should. If you are a man, consuming more than two drinks a day puts you at risk for high triglyceride levels. Women, on the other hand, shouldn't consume more than one drink if they want to keep their body lean and healthy.

High Blood Pressure. Those people who have hypertension (high blood pressure) are most likely to also have high triglyceride levels. If your blood pressure is high, regulating it with medication and a low-sodium diet may also help you knock down the triglycerides, if that is the only thing that elevates them, of course.

Type 2 Diabetes. Although having high triglycerides doesn't really seem to be a priority when you are struggling with high blood sugar, having this type of fat elevated can only worsen the overall health and shorten the path to heart diseases. Managing your diabetes regularly and following the dietary guidelines found in this book can also help you manage your triglyceride levels.

Medications. Sometimes, it is the thing that your doctor prescribes that can hurt your health. Some medications are known to have the power to increase the bad cholesterol and triglyceride levels. If you are consuming birth control pills, diuretics, or have been prescribed an estrogen therapy, these medications may be what triggers your triglycerides to sky-rocket. Check with your doctor and see if these medications are to blame for your high triglycerides, and if so, consult with them for a change in therapy.

Heredity. Sometimes, fat simply runs in the family. It is not uncommon for bad cholesterol and high triglycerides to be passed on. If these fat types are attributed to your family, it is possible that you have unfortunately inherited them. But don't worry. A dietary and lifestyle change may help you lower them. And this book will tell you exactly what you should eat to battle them once and for all.

Symptoms

The trickiest thing about having high triglycerides is the fact that they have no actual symptoms, meaning that there is no way for you to detect them on your own, unless they have caused some other complications.

Most people find out about their high triglyceride levels through a routing blood test. However, keep in mind that a simple cholesterol check doesn't necessarily mean that the triglyceride levels will also be measured.

Like I said, high triglyceride may only cause symptoms if they have contributed to some serious condition, such as coronary heart disease. In that case, the symptoms may include:

- Chest Pain

- Stroke

- Heart Attack

If you have extremely high triglyceride levels, there are some other things that you may notice:

- *Xanthomas* – cholesterol deposits that form below the skin under your eyes, and usually look something like yellow streaks

- Nodules on your knees and elbows

- Many skin eruptions that have the size of a pimple and are yellowish in color

The fact that they show no symptoms, until it's too late, is why The American Heart Association suggests that the triglyceride levels should be checked every 5 years after the age of 20.

Diagnosing

Detecting your triglyceride levels is a really simple process. Your doctor can easily determine them with a simple blood teste called lipid profile. Lipid profile is a blood test that measures your total cholesterol levels, the levels of your good HDL cholesterol, your bad LDL cholesterol, as well as the triglyceride levels.

This test is conducted after a 12-hour fasting period, for more accurate results. Since your triglyceride and cholesterol levels will most likely be higher after you eat, fasting is required if you want to see a clear picture of what's going on in your bloodstream.

Okay, but how high is too high? Here is how you can determine whether the levels of triglycerides in your blood fall into a normal range:

Normal – Less than 150 mg/dL or less than 1.7mmol/L

Borderline High – 150 to 199 mg/dL or 1.8 to 2.2 mmol/L

High – 200 to 499 milligrams per deciliter mg/dL or 2.3 to 5.6 mmol/L

Very High – 500mg/L or above or 5.7 mmol/L or more

There are also some other factors that may affect your triglyceride levels on the blood test results. Those include:

- Menstrual Cycle

- Blood Alcohol Levels
- Recent Exercise

Triglyceride to HDL Ratio

I have already mentioned that triglycerides have a tight relationship with the HDL (the good type) cholesterol. We know that the good cholesterol is important in getting rid of the oxidized particles of the bad LDL cholesterol that contribute to inflammation and disease of the arteries. Unfortunately, having high triglyceride levels usually coexists with having low HDL cholesterol levels. One of the important factors for seeing just how badly your triglyceride levels affect your health, is determining the triglyceride to HDL ratio.

This ratio is important because it considers the triglyceride and HDL levels in proportion to one another. That means that this ratio is an indicator of just how much the HDL cholesterol particles can balance out the pro-inflammatory particles of the triglycerides. Obviously, the ideal scenario would be a low triglyceride to HDL ratio, because that would mean a lower risk for inflammation or heart diseases. That ideal ratio is 1, meaning that the ideal balance between the triglyceride and HDL cholesterol is to have equal parts of them.

You'd think that high levels of HDL are better, which may be true, however, keep in mind that these levels rarely are higher than 100 mg/dL, and when they do, that is usually a sign that something is not functioning right. We said how healthy triglyceride levels are below 150 mg/dL. So, since the HDL don't go above 100 mg/dL, ideally, the triglyceride levels shouldn't either.

A healthy triglyceride to HDL ratio should be less than 2, but less than 3 is also satisfactory.

Unfortunately, as time goes by, it is more common to see people with rations 5:1. When the ratio is 7:1, it is dangerously high, and it is usually a sign that there is a serious health imbalance (such is the presence of diabetes or metabolic syndrome).

Risks of High Triglycerides

We usually do not pay as much attention to the triglycerides as we do to cholesterol, however, having high levels of triglycerides can be just as dangerous.

You have probably heard the expression "silent killer" referring to the high cholesterol levels. It shows absolutely no signs, but if left untreated, it can be fatal. Well, maybe the triglyceride levels don't harm with the same altitude as cholesterol, but if not managed, they can also contribute to some very threatening conditions:

Cardiovascular Diseases. Many studies have shown that elevated levels of triglycerides can indeed cause cardiovascular disease, which, unfortunately, is the primary cause of death in the Western countries. We often associate the heart disease with high cholesterol levels, but keep in mind that cardiovascular disease may indeed occur when the triglyceride levels are high, even if the levels of LDL cholesterol are not alarming at all.

A Harvard study from 2010 shows that having low HDL cholesterol and high triglyceride levels increases the odds for coronary heart disease, even after the LDL cholesterol has been reduced. This study has shown that the risk for a heart disease increases by 20% per 23 mg/dL of a triglyceride increase.

Diabetes. If you have high triglyceride levels, then you are more likely to develop a type 2 diabetes. No, I am not saying that having elevated triglycerides is what causes diabetes, but high triglycerides are a clear sign that the body is not burning enough fat, which means that the energy cannot be properly converted.

Having high triglycerides is usually tightly linked to a condition called metabolic syndrome or insulin resistance. Insulin is important for our body to transports the glucose to those cells that need energy, which means that the insulin is crucial for our body to convert the triglycerides into energy. And since being insulin resistant means having elevated triglyceride and vice versa, that will lead to a sugar build up in the bloodstream.

Pancreatitis. The pancreas is an organ found on the left side and upper part of the belly, that is of great importance for our overall health. It oversees producing digestive juices that help our gut absorb and digest the consumed food. Having very high triglyceride levels can, unfortunately, cause pancreas swelling. When the pancreas is swollen, it can no longer function properly. This may lead to fever, vomiting, and a severe abdominal pain. In some extreme situations, it can also contribute for the digestive juices to leak outside the pancreas, which is extremely dangerous and life-threatening. If you (or a loved one) have pancreatitis, the dietary changes, meal plan, and advice found in this book can help you treat that condition.

Stroke. Probably the most feared complication that can occur because of both increased triglycerides and cholesterol levels, is the restriction of the blood flow. High triglyceride levels can cause a plague in the arteries, which will lead to their hardening. In this condition, the arteries narrow and work as an obstacle for the blood. The flow of the blood is restricted, which means that the blood has a trouble to get to the heart and brain on time. This not only leads to heart attack but stroke as well.

High triglyceride levels can restrict the flow of blood within the vessels that should supply the brain cells with blood, which can lead to a brain damage called *stroke.*

Did you know that over 800,000 Americans have a stroke each year? This can be even more dangerous for you if you are a woman since recent studies show that elevated triglyceride levels are the number one risk factor for stroke for women.

Liver Disease. This one is obvious, isn't it? We said how the triglycerides that aren't used as an energy are stored inside the liver. Having high triglyceride levels means having excess fat accumulated inside the liver. This excess fat is anything but healthy and can lead to a chronic liver disease.

This disease can further leaf to permanent liver scarring, liver cancer, or a complete liver failure which can be life-threatening. In the fatty liver disease that is not caused by alcohol, approximately 10 percent of the liver is replaced with fat. The main causes for the NAFLD (non-alcoholic fatty liver disease) are high triglycerides, diabetes, and obesity.

PAD (Peripheral Artery Disease). If you have too much fat in your blood, which is what happens if you have high triglycerides, your blood is at a high risk for having deposits formed in. These deposits form in the arteries that flow to the legs, which leads to Peripheral Artery Disease (PAD). This is a condition that causes pain and numbness in the legs, which can be extremely inconvenient while walking. PAD increases the chance for developing a leg infection.

Dementia. We know that age is the main factor for developing dementia, however, what we don't know is that high triglycerides can also be a very strong risk factor. Dementia is a condition that results in loss of the brain function. That can affect your thinking, memory, language, and overall behavior. Many studies have proven that high triglycerides can not only damage the blood vessels in the brain but also contribute to the toxic protein called *amyloid* to get piled up inside.

Changing the Unhealthy Lifestyle

Fortunately for all of you whose blood test results show elevated triglyceride levels, most of the risk factors that lead to the increase in triglycerides are very much changeable. Even if you are old or if high triglyceride runs in your family, you can still keep them at bay by adopting a much healthier diet and changing your lifestyle for the better.

The focus of this book is, of course, the diet that leads to the drop in triglyceride levels. However, I would be lying if I told you that re-stocking your fridge and pantry with healthy ingredients is the magic bullet for a healthy heart. The dietary guidelines found in this book cannot help you lower your high triglyceride if you don't commit to a whole lifestyle change, first.

Be Active

Although this one shouldn't need any explanation, it seems that it is the most alarming one of all. Being inactive and not burning any calories results in fat build-up on your belly, hips, and thighs, and with that a raise in the triglyceride levels.

We are all aware of how beneficial physical activity can be for our overall health, but not everyone knows that it can contribute to lowering the triglyceride levels. And I am not only talking about the obvious fat-burning, weight-loss contribution. Even though regular exercise can help you burn fat and lower the triglycerides, there are also two very important ways in which physical activity can help you knock down the triglyceride levels:

1. Regular exercise can stimulate the enzymes that are in charge of transferring the triglycerides and LDL cholesterol to the liver.

2. Physical activity can also enlarge the size of the lipoproteins that carry the cholesterol and triglycerides through the bloodstream.

If all of this seems too overwhelming, know that you don't have to sign up for a marathon to lower your triglycerides. Some simple activities like walking around the block, doing more household chores, jogging for 15 minutes, etc. can all contribute to the triglyceride drop.

Say "No" to the Refill

If you thought that I would suggest total alcohol abstinence, here are some good news. Alcohol consumption is not only allowed, but it is also encouraged. Only if you are not thinking about refilling the glass, that is.

We are often alarmed about frequent alcohol consumption and it seems that the warning signs are everywhere. However, The National Institute of Health (NIH) is against complete abstinence. When it is consumed in moderation (which is no more than 2 drinks a day for men and 1 drink for women), alcohol can in fact decrease the blood clotting, and even raise the HDL cholesterol levels. If it is consumed frequently, and in larger amounts, alcohol will increase the triglyceride levels. A healthified low-cholesterol and low-triglyceride diet will do you no good if you choose to destroy your balanced meals with a couple of drinks.

If you can say "No" to the refill, there is no need for you to be the party breaker.

Stop Smoking

If you are one of those people that have been justifying their smoking with the fact that they are not gaining weight, well, let me tell you how wrong you are. If you are a smoker that has tried to quit smoking, then you know what I am talking about. What is the easiest way to satisfy your urge when you don't want to smoke? Food, of course. That is why when people give up smoking, they usually gain a few pounds. If you think that smoking is better than carrying the fat and triglycerides around your tummy, know that it is not.

Even if you gain some weight after you stop smoking, you will still have lower triglycerides than if you do not gain the weight but smoke regularly. One study conducted by the University of Wisconsin have found that those people who stop smoking increase their HDL cholesterol levels and can also experience a drop in the triglycerides, lower LDL cholesterol levels, as well as positive changes in the lipids.

Yes, it is addictive, and yes, it is hard to quit, I will not lie. However, thinking about the long term, wouldn't you rather reach a hale and hearty retirement than experiencing a stroke before your time?

The average smoker quits 6 times before finally giving up smoking. Do not lose faith!

Choosing the Right Diet

Low-carb or low-fat? It seems that the nutritionists cannot make up their minds about what it seems to be the never-ending debate in the world of health and nutrition. Should you really choose a full-fat milk and bacon to lose weight and lower the triglyceride and cholesterol? Or should you stick to the well-known low-calorie approach and consume fewer calories, choosing the nonfat options for getting rid of the fat? The ladder seems kind of obvious, but is it true?

If you have spent some time googling "High Triglyceride Diet" or "Low Cholesterol Diet", then you have stumbled upon split opinions and contradictory theories. And to make it even more confusing, there are actual studies backing up both low-carb and low-fat diets. But which one is the smartest choice?

It is indeed true that the low-carb diets, such as the Ketogenic diet, have shown some extraordinary results in burning fat, even though it is a high-fat diet, however, you need to keep in mind that the research, studies, and the scientific back-up that this diet has is limited. There is simply lack of evidence that shows that the low-carb diets are best for reducing the cholesterol and triglyceride levels, so I wouldn't bet my life on it.

But that doesn't mean that you should go all crazy and track every single morsel that goes into your mouth to lower the calorie intake. What's important is to steer clear of the forbidden food items (see next chapter) and enrich your diet with healthy fats instead.

Go Mediterranean

No, I am not talking about going on a cruise around the Mediterranean (although who wouldn't want that, right?). I am talking about choosing one of the healthiest diets ever. I am pretty sure that most of you are aware of this, but when it comes to having a healthy heart, there is no better diet than the Mediterranean diet.

The Mediterranean diet is a diet that is present in the countries that surround the Mediterranean Sea and is especially present in Greece and southern Italy. The diet emphasizes the consumption of healthy fats, lean meats plenty of fruits and vegetables, whole grains, and nuts. There are many studies that have conducted that people who live in these countries have a lower incidence of developing a cardiovascular disease compared to other population outside of the Mediterranean region.

But that is not all. Apparently, the Mediterranean diet is successful is lowering the risk of cancer and other chronic diseases, and the thing that we are most concerned with today – it has also been proven that it can lower the triglycerides and bad cholesterol levels.

21

If you are looking for a study that can back this up, know that there are plenty. All these studies have concluded that the Mediterranean diet is perhaps the best heart-healthy diet there is. This is thanks to the fact that this diet is effective at lowering the lipid levels, increasing the HDL cholesterol, and decreasing the level of triglycerides. Most studies have also found that the Mediterranean diet can also lower the oxidation of the bad LDL cholesterol. And if that's not good enough, know that this diet can also lower the blood pressure, blood sugar, and even the incidence of asthma.

The Mediterranean diet is packed with triglyceride and cholesterol friendly ingredients and emphasizes the consumption of polyunsaturated fat. The polyunsaturated fat is the best type of fatty acid since it can lead to regulation of the triglycerides and cholesterol. And the Mediterranean diet is jam-packed with it. It focuses on the high consumption of nuts, seeds, seafood, olive oil (all polyunsaturated fats), and restrict the intake of processed meat, processed foods, and sugars. This makes this diet superior to other low-fat diets and even more beneficial than the popular low-carb diets, even though it doesn't restrict the consumption of complex carbohydrates.

The Mediterranean diet is balanced, not very restrictive, and easy to follow. It consists of:

- Foods high in the healthy fats such as seeds, nuts, and olive oil

- High-fiber grains such as oats, barley, quinoa, wild rice, millet, etc.

- Lean cuts of meat. More poultry and lower consumption of red meat.

- Moderate consumption of seafood, especially fish that is high in omega-3 fatty acids such as salmon, mackerel, anchovy, etc.

- Plenty fresh fruits and veggies

- Low to moderate consumption of dairy products

- Foods that are high in phytosterols such as nuts and legumes.

It is flexible, easy to follow, and heart healthy. However, you must keep in mind that the Mediterranean diet is not actually designed for the decrease of the triglycerides. Sure, it can help you regulate them and restore balance in your bloodstream which will contribute to the health of your heart, but you need to be aware that it isn't the magical cure. Once you manage to lower your triglycerides – after restricting all the foods that may trigger them – you may go full Mediterranean to keep them in check. Until that happens, you will need to pay a little bit more attention to your plates than simply avoiding the processed food. The next chapter will help you understand exactly what needs to be purged out of your kitchen.

What Not to Eat

Triglycerides may not receive the same degree of attention as cholesterol does but having a high level of them can indeed hurt your health, and in extreme situations, it can also be fatal. But don't let this scare you. Having a blood test result that shows elevated triglycerides can be alarming, but it can also be easily managed.

The first thing that you need to take care of after finding that you have more than the recommended amount of triglycerides in your blood, is to get rid of all the triggers. You may be used to eating junk food and drowning in bowls of ice cream (which is most likely why your triglyceride levels have skyrocketed in the first place), but if you want to regulate the fat in your body, dietary changes are not required but crucial.

Below you will see a list of what should be excluded from your diet completely, to regulate the triglycerides. Make sure that your diet will be free of these triggers, and you have nothing to worry about.

Sugar. It seems that no matter how much we are warned about the side effects of sugar; this sweet hazard still ends up in our tummies. Its addicting nature makes it hard for us to shake off our

24

sugar cravings, but when we are staring at a possible heart problem, we better say no to the sweet stuff.

I say sugar, but I do not only mean the white granules that you add in your desserts and coffee. Sugar comes in many forms and has multiple disguises. Make sure to avoid:

- White Sugar

- Brown Sugar

- Coconut Sugar

- Honey

- Maple Syrup

- Agave Nectar

- Fructose

- Corn Syrup

- Molasses

- Date Sugar

- Birch Syrup

All the above are forms of sugar. They will not only increase your triglyceride levels an amount of fat in your body but can also drag a list of other potential health risks. When grocery shopping, make sure to read the labels well to ensure that there are no hidden sugars.

Be careful! Just because the label may say "no added sugar" or "sugar-free", that does not mean that it will not raise your triglycerides. This is especially the case for fruity drinks and snacks that are packed with fructose. To be safe, avoid buying juices and other foods made from fruit. The Cleveland Clinic recommends choosing fresh fruit instead of buying juices.

Natural sugar found in ingredients that are higher in carbs can also have a negative impact on your triglycerides. Make sure to limit the consumption of starchy foods such as beans, peas, and potatoes, and not consume more than 2/3 cup per day. Dried fruit can be beneficial, but only if it is restricted to ¼ cup per day.

Refined Carbohydrates. Refined carbohydrates are the easiest way to pack yourself with energy, because they are broken down into glucose fast. That may sound like a good thing, but it is not. Also called simple carbohydrates, the refined carbs provide with fast, but short-lasting energy, usually followed by a crash.

Refined carbohydrates such as bread, pasta, bagels, and tortillas that are made from white flour, have a high glycemic index, which means that consuming refined grains does not only increases your blood sugar, but the triglyceride and cholesterol levels as well.

Know that your body converts the simple carbs into triglycerides. Also, given the fact that these carbs lose their fiber intake during the refining process, they hold absolutely no health benefits whatsoever. Make sure to avoid:

- Refined Grains such as white rice

- Foods made with white flour

- Enriched or bleached flours and foods made with them

Processed Meat. Studies have shown that processed meats are strongly associated with the increase of triglycerides and cholesterol, and that they can contribute to the development of cardiovascular diseases. Processed meats have more than 50 percent higher sodium content than the unprocessed meat, which makes them not only bad for our triglycerides and cholesterol, but overall health as well.

Make sure to avoid:

- Bacon

- Salami

- Sausages

- Ham

- Corned Beef

- Prosciutto

- Corn Dogs

- Fish sticks and patties

- Meat jerky

- Lunch meats

Trans Fats. They are fats that are healthy and then there are those that are fat in the true sense of the word. The trans fats are just like that. They are partially hydrogenated oils that are made with the sole purpose of adding them to food to give them a better texture and taste. However, beside that they can improve the taste and flavor, the trans fats can hurt your health. Foods that are high in trans fats can easily raise your triglyceride and cholesterol levels. Avoid eating:

- Vegetable and processed oils

- French fries and deep-fried foods

- Chips

- Donuts

- Prepackaged baked goods like pie crusts and pizza crusts

- Other packaged foods

Butter. You may think that avoiding butter is impossible since pretty much everything is made with it. However, since you should focus more on home cooked meals and avoid eating dishes that you don't know the full ingredient list off, I say ditching butter, or the sake of your regulated triglycerides can be simple.

Butter is rich in trans and saturated fats which are the main contributors to the increase of your triglyceride levels. But don't think that substituting butter with other shortenings such as margarine is a healthier option. Margarine is also packed with the bad types of fat and should also be avoided.

Ghee. So, let's just swap the butter with ghee, then, right? Although there are diets that recommend the consumption of ghee, this clarified butter can be equally unfriendly to your triglycerides. Many studies have found that ghee, thanks to its rich palmitic acid content, can contribute to the clogging of the arteries. Besides, clarified butter is just as high in saturated fat which can only raise your LDL and triglyceride levels.

Liver. So, you've heard that eating liver can help you boost your hemoglobin. It is true that liver can provide benefits to some aspects of your health thanks to its rich iron content. However, your triglyceride level is not one of those aspects.

It may help you boost your iron, but it will also increase your triglycerides and the bad LDL cholesterol. Liver, as well as any organs for that matter (brain, heart, sweetbreads, etc.), should be avoided by people that have elevated triglyceride or cholesterol levels.

Coconut. Coconut may be trendy these days since it seems that all the popular diets swear by its magical benefits. However, if you are struggling with increased triglycerides, coconut shouldn't be an ingredient found in your kitchen. Coconut is high in saturated fats and as such it can easily raise your triglycerides and cholesterol. You can consult with your doctor and see if it is safe for you to consume coconut, and if so, how much. If your doctor thinks that there is no need for you to limit it, you can choose low-fat options to further limit the saturated fat consumptions.

Before your doctor gives you a green light (in case they do so), it is safer for you to stay away from coconut and all coconut products:

- Coconut flakes
- Coconut oil
- Coconut milk
- Coconut cream

Whole-Fat Dairy. You have probably heard how milk and dairy products contain a broad range of different fatty acids. Well, some of those fatty acids can have a pretty negative effect on those lipoproteins that are rich in cholesterol. Lauric acid and myristic acid are especially negative since they can increase the total plasma cholesterol, and with that your triglycerides and the bad LDL cholesterol. High in calories and saturated fatty acids, the

29

conventional full-fat dairy products can easily increase your triglycerides.

But that doesn't mean that you should completely avoid dairy. Dairy can provide your health with other nutrients that can be beneficial. If you choose low-fat dairy products you can still receive these benefits without worrying about your triglycerides or cholesterol.

Fatty Meats. The fat found in the animal meat is saturated fat. And since we know that the saturated fat is only good for raising our triglycerides and LDL cholesterol, you should make sure that you will not buy any fatty cuts of meat to avoid getting your triglycerides spiked.

Canned Fish in Oil. Fish is super beneficial for pretty much every aspect of your health, triglycerides included. However, when it comes to buying canned fish, you should be extra careful. The best way for you to ensure that you will up your omega-3 fatty acids without worrying that the fat from the oil will raise your triglycerides and cholesterol is to buy only canned fish in water, not oil. It is common for the canned fish to be packed in oil that is rich in saturated oil, so make sure to avoid that.

The Egg, Meat, and Shellfish Myth

Talk to a couple of different nutritionists and you will get different opinions regarding the triglycerides and overall cholesterol. Doctors, too. Some may prescribe medications right away, while others will tell you that nothing but a strict diet is required for you to regulate the triglycerides.

Don't get me wrong. I am not a doctor and I am most certainly not qualified to give you medical advice regarding your own unique health condition. However, what I do know are the facts. And there are many facts about the diet that should lower the triglycerides and cholesterol that are confusing.

Eggs or no eggs? Red meat or no red meat? Shellfish or only fish? The opinions are split, and the recommendations are confusing, to say the least. So how to know who's right and who's not? Here is what you should know about eggs, red meat, and shellfish.

Eggs

The fact that eggs are high in cholesterol is undeniable. In the United States, most of the dietary cholesterol, as well as elevated triglycerides, comes from eggs and dishes made with eggs. *Conclusion*: eggs increase the LDL cholesterol and triglycerides.

31

But eggs are a real powerhouse. They are packed with antioxidant properties that can help you lower the risk of developing a heart disease   and   cancer. *Conclusion:* eggs are good for your heart.

Eggs are good for your heart, but triglycerides and cholesterol aren't. You see how this can be confusing?

The cholesterol in the eggs is mostly found in the yolks, which means that eating egg yolks can increase the triglyceride and cholesterol, not eating egg whites. There is no need for you to ditch eggs completely. You can safely consume egg whites without worrying about your triglycerides. But, since the yolks can be extremely beneficial for your health, you shouldn't avoid them completely. Incorporating a whole egg here and there can be healthy, if you limit the yolk consumption.

Red Meat

The myth about red meat is in the fact that this type of meat is higher than saturated fats. But not all red meat is the same. And while it is true that red meat is fattier than poultry, it is a well-known fact that eating lean red meat is quite beneficial, and there are many studies that can back this up. Omitting red meat altogether is not a good approach for lowering the triglyceride levels. Instead, you should avoid the fatty cuts of meat (as mentioned in the previous chapter) and focus on the leaner cuts. Eat lean red meat in moderation.

When buying red meat makes sure that it is grass fed, and 100% organic. Do not buy "prime" meat, as that means that the meat is higher in saturated fats.

Shellfish

Shellfish may be higher in cholesterol than regular fish, however, that is not a reason for you to ditch the multiple benefits and healthy fatty acids that shellfish are packed with. Eating shrimp and scallops here and there can be quite beneficial for your health. If you do not overdo it and make lobster a regular meal (one ounce of lobster contains 20 mg of cholesterol), there is no need for you to completely avoid eating shellfish.

Foods that Lower Triglycerides

Just like there are foods that are high in unhealthy fats and that can increase your triglyceride and cholesterol, there are also those foods that are packed with healthy properties that can help you lower the amount of these fat types in your blood.

Having elevated triglyceride levels in your blood may force you to say farewell to eating junk food and butter-drowned fatty meats, however, that does not mean that you should eat nothing but leafy greens.

Here are some foods that are low in cholesterol and that can help you battle the high triglycerides.

Vegetables. Although I have mentioned that veggies that are high in starchy content and are rich in carbs should be consumed in moderation, know that absolutely all vegetables are a welcome addition to your High Triglyceride Diet. It is recommended to eat 3 to 5 servings of vegetables per day to lower your triglycerides and LDL cholesterol.

The best choices include:

Spinach. Spinach is not only beneficial to improve your iron content and pack you with super amazing antioxidant properties. Spinach is also rich in lutein (over 11.000 mg in only 100 grams of spinach), which is super helpful for preventing the clogging of the arteries, which can happen because of high triglycerides and LDL cholesterol. It can also assist your triglyceride lowering goal, so making spinach a regular part of your diet is more than recommended.

Not only spinach is beneficial. All leafy greens can, in fact, help you lower your triglycerides in one way or another. And the best part? It's almost as they have no calories, so feel free to consume them as much as you want.

Tomatoes. Tomatoes are packed with an amazing property called lycopene, and many studies have found that lycopene is helpful at lowering the triglycerides and cholesterol. In fact, eating lycopene-rich tomatoes can help you lower the unhealthy fats from your blood by 10 percent in just a couple of weeks. And that is just by implementing tomatoes into your diet. But that's not the best part. What's even more amazing is that tomatoes are even richer in lycopene when they are cooked. If that's not a reason for you to cook your own pasta sauce, I don't know what is.

Garlic. Although some will argue that garlic is an herb, I believe it should be listed under this category. Wearing the crown for the most heart-healthy ingredients (which is also the most well-researched ingredient as well), this anti-inflammatory, anti-viral, antioxidant, and immune-boosting ingredient can also lower your triglyceride levels, lower the LDL cholesterol, prevent your arteries from clogging, as well as knock down your blood pressure. If you don't like eating it on its own, implement garlic as much as you can in marinades, soups, sauces, salads, and when roasting veggies.

Eggplants and Okra. Both eggplants and okra are excellent choices of soluble fiber, are low in calories and can help you lower the triglyceride levels. Make sure to implement them into your diet whenever you see fit.

Sweet Potatoes. Providing loads of antioxidants and vitamins along with some good artery-cleansing fiber, sweet potatoes are not only low in calories, but they also have a low glycemic index. Implementing sweet potatoes into your diet can help you knock down your triglycerides.

Other great vegetables that can help you lower the high triglyceride levels are:

- Onions
- Brussel Sprouts
- Asparagus
- Butternut Squash
- Broccoli
- Bell Peppers
- Cauliflower
- Cabbage
- Artichokes
- Carrots
- Mushrooms
-

Fruits. Eating fresh fruits can be more than beneficial for reducing the fat content from your bloodstream. However, since they are higher in fructose, you should pay attention not to overdo it. They are healthy and helpful for regulating triglycerides, but if you choose to make fruit the star of your meals, they will do nothing but support weight gain.

There are many types of fruit that can help you lower the triglycerides. The most beneficial ones are:

Avocados. Of course, how can a healthy diet lack avocado? Rich in the healthiest monounsaturated fats, avocados are the staple of any diet. That said, avocados are perhaps the greatest source of the healthy fats that contribute to heart health. Besides, eating only ½ avocado a day can significantly improve your HDL cholesterol, lower the LDL cholesterol, and in turn, cause a drop in our triglyceride levels.

Packed with soluble fiber, avocados can also help you balance your blood sugar and pack you with anti-inflammatory phytochemicals that will help you keep the high triglycerides at bay.

But that is not all. Avocados are also rich in Niacin (Vitamin B3) that lower the production of triglycerides and bad cholesterol, and contributes to the process of their elimination, as well. Best sources of niacin, besides avocados, are veggies like potatoes, asparagus, corn, mushrooms, and artichokes.

Citrus Fruits. If you love drinking orange juice in the morning, here is some good news. Oranges – and all citrus fruits – can help you lower the triglyceride levels and boost the good HDL cholesterol. Thanks to their high vitamin C content, citrus fruits contribute to preventing the cholesterol oxidation. Their high anti-oxidant properties content will help you regulate your overall blood picture.

Other fruits that are high in vitamin C are:

- Strawberries

- Mango

- Pineapple

- Passionfruit

Berries. We know how rich in anti-oxidants berries are, but how can they help you lower the triglyceride levels? Berries, especially blueberries, blackberries, and cranberries, have a high content of vitamin E, which prevents the growth of plagues in the blood vessels. That means that berries, and vitamin E in general, keep the arteries healthy and 'clean' and prevent the triglycerides from piling up in the blood.

Other foods that contain vitamin E that you should consume for lowering the triglyceride levels are:

- Guava

- Kiwi

- Mango

- Nectarines and Peaches

- Papaya

Apples. Apples – especially their skin – are loaded with pectin, which is a type of soluble fiber that can latch itself onto the triglycerides and bad LDL cholesterol, and then guide their way through our gut and then out of our body. This effectively lowers the triglyceride levels, LDL cholesterol, and respectively improves the triglyceride to HDL ratio. Citrus fruits are also packed with the pectin, but keep in mind that it is mostly found in their pulp. To get your pectin dose from citrus, you will have to eat the fruit, not drink the juice.

Besides apples and citrus fruits, other fruits that ate rich in soluble fiber are:

- Pears

- Berries

- Apricots

- Prunes

- Figs

-

Fish. Eating fish that is rich in the anti-inflammatory omega-3 fatty acids can help you significantly boost your HDL cholesterol and with that improve your triglyceride to HDL ratio. And while there is a lack of studies that show the direct way in which fish can lower your triglycerides and bad LDL cholesterol, it is a well-known fact that the omega threes are indeed linked to low rates of heart diseases, low blood pressure, and many other conditions.

The best sources of omega-3 fatty acids are:

- Salmon

- Mackerel

- Tuna

- Sardines

-

Nuts. And you thought that there wasn't a healthy and crunchy snack. Nuts, of all kinds really, are a great source of monounsaturated and polyunsaturated fats. And since we have mentioned a couple of times before how great these fats are for lowering the triglycerides and boosting the HDL cholesterol, you can only imagine how beneficial munching on nuts can be for your health.

Nuts also provide a significant amount of fiber, which is an added plus. Studies show that nuts are great at preventing artery damages and protect our blood vessels from the triglyceride and cholesterol buildup. This also happens thanks to their flavonoid content – a plant-based antioxidant compound that reduce inflammation and improve our artery health.

Almonds, pecans, macadamia nuts, cashews, peanuts, hazelnuts, are all good choices. The only thing you need to keep an eye on is the portion size. Nuts are known to be richer in calories, so make sure not to consume more than a couple of ounces a day. That is enough for you to reap all the benefits without increasing the calorie consumption.

Seeds. Being one of the main food types in the Mediterranean diet, seeds are also great at improving not only the health of the heart, but our overall health as well. And the best part? Studies have proven that they are also amazing at lowering the unhealthy fats from our blood.

Although all kinds of seeds are great: sesame seeds, sunflower seeds, pumpkin seeds, etc. when it comes to lowering our triglyceride levels, the seeds that we should pack our diet the most are flaxseeds and chia seeds.

They are the richest sources of the plant-based ALA (alpha-linolenic acid) which is a type of omega three fatty acid that is super powerful at fighting off inflammation. Chia seeds and flaxseeds are high in both, soluble and insoluble fiber. They are great at trapping the cholesterol and triglycerides in the digestive system, making it harder for our body to absorb them. All in all, their contribution to the decrease of triglycerides and cholesterol is amazing.

Whole Grains. 100 % whole grains are the best source of fiber. And since fiber is a very important factor in the process of lowering triglycerides and cholesterol, it is obvious how helpful it is to eat whole grains.

Oats. Oats are packed with a substance that is called *beta-glucan* which is a substance that tends to absorb the unhealthy fats from the blood. Ever wondered what causes oats to bulk up in liquid? Well, that is the soluble fiber called beta-glucan. Just like they can absorb the liquid, the oats can also absorb cholesterol (the bad kind) and triglycerides. This compound forms a sticky layer in your small intestine which blocks these fats from getting into your bloodstream
Make oatmeal a healthy and regular breakfast choice. Combine it with fruits such as apples or berries, seeds, and nuts, and boost up the soluble fiber even more.

Quinoa. Just like oats, quinoa is also rich in soluble fiber. This ancient and protein-rich grain contributes to the health of your heart by lowering the triglycerides and cholesterol. So, what happens when you eat quinoa? The soluble fiber from the quinoa combines with your liver's bile acids and create an excretion that is jelly-like. The liver's bile acids are created with the stored unhealthy fats. So, when the fiber of the quinoa takes some of that bile acid, your liver is forced to take some more fats to create it. The more bile acids are created, the lower the level of bad fats such as LDL cholesterol and triglycerides. Conclusion: the more quinoa you eat, the lower the level of the unhealthy fats in your blood.

When it comes to whole grains, the accent should be put on the gluten-free types such as oats, quinoa, buckwheat, amaranth, etc. Gluten-free grains are much easier to digest and do not promote inflammation. However, gluten whole-grains can also be beneficial. Thinks brown and wild rice. These grains can give your health a powerful kick as well, so I do not recommend excluding them from your diet completely. Make sure to include ½ cup of cooked whole-grain rice and barley, here and there.

Beans and Legumes. We all know that beans are healthy due to their high fiber content and complex carbohydrates. However, what you may not know is that beans and legumes can help you lower your triglyceride levels:

- They are high in soluble fiber which can help you lower the LDL cholesterol and triglyceride levels, by slowing the amount and rate of absorption of these fats.

- They are an amazing source of resistant starch, which is another way in which can help you lower the triglycerides.

- They are high in phytosterols which is a plant-based cholesterol that can help you lower the cholesterol.

- They are rich in antioxidants and other trace minerals that support a healthy circulation, keep the triglycerides balanced, and support your heart health.

They are amazing, but don't go for one kind only. Try them all if you can: kidney beans, pinto beans, black beans, chickpeas, mung beans, lentils, etc. Use them in soups, salads, veggie patties, and of course, don't forget the good old hummus.

Olive Oil. You couldn't possibly go Mediterranean if olive oil is not a huge part of your diet. Being rich in heart-healthy and extremely beneficial monounsaturated fats, olive oil can indeed help you lower your high triglycerides. There are other healthy oil choices such as Flaxseed oil or avocado oil, but even though flaxseeds and avocados can help you lower your triglycerides, their oils cannot do the same as olive oil. Olive oil is beyond doubt the king of all oils. It has the highest concentration of monounsaturated fats, and with that can lower the risk of the artery clogging and heart disease.

Make sure to make olive oil the staple of your diet. Just remember, there isn't a limit. But do not only use it for cooking and salads. Try to drizzle all your meals with olive oil. You can even take pieces of whole wheat pita bread and dunk it in olive oil and spices.

Dark Chocolate. If you are a chocolate lover (and who isn't?) then you will love to hear that eating chocolate can improve your triglyceride levels and overall health. Okay, not the sugar-packed milk chocolate, but dark chocolate can lower your triglycerides.

Dark chocolate and cocoa powder (the unsweetened kind), both contain flavonoids. Flavonoids are a powerful antioxidant that can help you lower your LDL cholesterol and triglyceride levels by reducing the oxidation of the LDL and preventing the platelets from joining forces. Studies have shown that flavonoids can increase the blood flow, relax the arterial muscles and lower the LDL cholesterol, triglycerides, and high blood pressure.

Flavonoids can also be found in other types of foods (green tea and red wine have these antioxidants), however, know that dark chocolate is packed with it. It contains three times the amount of flavonoids found in green tea, and twice the amount of these antioxidants that are found in red wine. And that is after most of the flavonoids that cacao is naturally packed with, are extracted due to the process of production of dark chocolate (that's where the bitter flavor comes from).

Green Tea. It may contain three times fewer flavonoids than dark chocolate, but thanks to the fact that it is practically calorie-free and that is packed with other antioxidant and anti-inflammatory properties, green tea should be a part of the high triglyceride diet. It prevents the triglyceride and cholesterol level from rising, it supports the heart health, it has anti-aging properties and it is known to be packed with cancer-fighting properties. If that's not a reason to swap your morning coffee for a cup of green tea, I don't know what is.

Kimchi. You may find this odd, but this Korean fermented side dish can help you lower your cholesterol levels. Made from radishes, cabbage, and cucumbers, Kimchi has been known for providing many health benefits, and lowering the unhealthy fats is just one of the many. Due to its beneficial bacteria (that is produced during the fermentation process), kimchi does not only keep your whole gut healthy, but it can also block the LDL cholesterol and triglycerides from being absorbed into our bloodstream.

If you are not a radish fan and do not like Kimchi, then perhaps *sauerkraut* is a great substitute. However, whether eating sauerkraut or kimchi, you need to be careful about the portion size. They are both loaded with sodium which can hurt your health in many other ways.

Turmeric. We have all heard that turmeric is the king of spices. When it comes to the health benefits and fighting the inflammation, that is. Containing an active ingredient called curcumin, it has been scientifically proven that including turmeric in your diet can protect you against many diseases such as heart disease, arthritis, and even cancer. And if that doesn't convince you to sprinkle turmeric on your dishes, perhaps the fact that it can lower cholesterol and triglycerides, will. Turmeric keeps our blood clean from the unhealthy fats and prevents its clogging.

Don't know how to increase your turmeric intake? Enjoy baked sweet potatoes sprinkled with turmeric, roasted turmeric chickpeas, add a few tablespoons when making creamy soups, add to your hummus, sprinkle over salads, etc.

Cooking Tips

It is not just what you eat. It is how you eat it that also matters. It is pointless to eat a bowl of broccoli if you boil them more than you should and lose all the important nutrients in the process. It will not hurt your health, but it will not improve it either.

When it comes to watching your triglyceride levels, it is extremely important for you to be aware not only of what you prepare, but how you prepare the food as well. You may not know this but choosing the allowed ingredients only isn't enough for you to lower your triglycerides. You will also need to pay close attention to how you will cook them as well.

When it comes to lowering the high triglycerides, or cholesterol in general, there are a couple of cooking rules that you need to be aware of. Some of these may be obvious to you, while some may be even life-changing. Be as it may, make sure to follow these rules to support the decrease of unhealthy fats from your blood.

Do NOT Boil – Steam Instead

When boiling veggies, almost all the beneficial nutrients that the veggies are packed with, get released into the cooking water.

Eating boiled asparagus will not provide you with the beneficial niacin that you can lower your triglycerides with. The only way you can consume the nutrients when boiling, is if you are making a soup or if you are about to consume the cooking liquid as well.

When looking for a way to cook veggies to serve alongside your fish or lean meat, the best way to prepare them is by steaming. Steaming your veggies is the only way for the food to preserve its nutrients. Instead of being drowned in boiling water, cooking them on steam will stop them from leeching the healthy nutrients out.

Do NOT Peel Fruits and Veggies

We all know that most of the nutrients of the fruits and veggies are found in the peel. Remember what we said about the peel of the apple? It contains more pectin (a type of soluble fiber that can lower your triglycerides and cholesterol) than the fruit itself. So, peeling an apple is not really recommended if you want to drop the triglycerides. But this doesn't apply only to apples. You shouldn't peel any fruit or vegetable if the peel is edible.

You may not know this, but the peel of the orange is packed with anti-cholesterol and anti-triglyceride properties. And while eating an orange peel is certainly neither tasty nor recommended, you can get the most of this fruit by grating the orange peel and sprinkling it over salads to provide yourself with yet another anti-triglyceride weapon.

Try not to peel eggplants and sweet potatoes as well, as they too are packed with healthy compounds that can assist you in your triglyceride decrease journey.

Wash the Fat Off

Do you know that you can wash the fat off your meat? Well, you cannot wash the fat off a fatty meat cut entirely, of course, but this is yet another way in which you can lower your saturated fat intake. And here is how you can do it:

- Chop your meat and place it in a pot filled with water.

- Cook it until the meat reaches the desired consistency.

- Place the meat in a strainer and pour boiling water over (clean water, not the cooking liquid).

- Pour boiling water once (or twice) more.

Rinsing the meat in boiling water may seem simple and honestly, too good to be true, but it works. You can not only cut back on the fat significantly, but this way your meat will have approximately 100 calories less. Amazing, right?

De-Skin Poultry

Most of the fat of the poultry is found in the skin. If you want to lower your triglyceride levels, you should de-skin the poultry. But, I do not mean to remove the skin after cooking, but cooking without the skin, since the fat from the skin can easily get transferred to the meat as well.

Keep in mind though, the de-skinning your meat will not make such a big difference if you fail to follow the other cooking tips.

Do NOT Fry

If you want to cut back on trans fats and saturated fats, then frying your food is not an option. Roast, grill, bake, or grill, but do not fry. Roast your veggies for a better flavor instead of frying them. Do not fry our meat on the stovetop, but place under a broiler and cook to perfection. Let it drain on the rack. If you want to make a gravy, make it with other ingredients such as red wine, juices or a healthy marinade. Always discard the drippings after cooking as they are packed with fats that can only increase your triglycerides.

Cook a Day Earlier

Cooking one day earlier will allow you to simply remove the fat. Whether boiled meat, soups, stocks, or stews, if you are planning to cook the fat in liquid, you can simply remove it by choosing to cook it one day ahead. Prepare your dish one day earlier and place in the fridge. The next day, you will see that most of the fat is visible and hardened on the top. Simply grab a spoon and remove it. That way you can significantly lower the fat content of the dish and not let your meal affect your triglyceride levels in a bad way.

Be Careful with the Oil

The only type of oil you should use is olive oil, period. Whether for cooking or drizzling over salads. However, olive oil does not work like other cooking oils. The best way for you to keep your meals safe while cooking is not to cook over 250 degrees F. Above this temperature, the oil will not only break the beneficial fatty acids and stop being helpful to your health, but it will also start to smoke.

My advice: do not fry. Use the oil for grilling, baking, broiling, roasting. Frying with olive oil on high temperature is not beneficial, so make sure that you will use the most of your oil.

Bake with Applesauce

Many baking recipes call for a butter, so if you think that you must skip eating healthy cakes and baked goods just because you are not allowed any, you are wrong. What butter does for the dough or batter, the same thing can applesauce or other pureed fruits do. Try including bananas in bread and muffins, use applesauce for oatmeal cookies and muffins also, try incorporating zucchini in brownies, etc.

Increase the Fiber

Like I said many, many times before, fiber is extremely helpful for your high triglycerides, as it can guide these unhealthy fats out of your body. That said, increasing the fiber intake seems like a pretty obvious thing to do. These simple tricks can help you do just that:

- To make breadcrumbs or croutons, just toast whole-grain bread and then crush or cube it.

- Although toasted breadcrumbs are better, breadcrumbs, in general, aren't that beneficial. See to substitute them with other whole grains where you see fit. For instance, when making meatballs or meatloaf, use uncooked oatmeal instead.

- Eat the rainbow. To ensure a proper fiber intake, you will have to eat as many colors of fruits and veggies as possible. When making salads, make sure you have lots of different colors (for instance, leafy greens, tomatoes, yellow bell pepper, onion, red cabbage, beets, etc.)

- Make sure that the flour you use is whole-wheat. An even better option would be to switch to baking with almond flour instead. Coconut flour is very popular, however, remember that coconut increases the triglycerides, so you should avoid it.

-

21-Day Meal Plan

Now that we have covered pretty much everything there is for you to know about lowering the triglycerides, it is time for me to present you a simple 21-day meal plan that can help you get started into a diet without the unhealthy fats.

There may be more planning involved, however, keep in mind that consuming a diet that is rich in low-cholesterol foods that lower the triglyceride levels is neither tasteless nor overwhelming.

Here is how you can use most of the allowed ingredients.

Day 1:

Breakfast:

1 cup of Oatmeal made with nonfat Milk
1 tablespoon of Raisins
1 tbsp Flaxseed
1 Tangerine

Snack 1:

A handful of Blackberries
½ cup nonfat Yogurt

Lunch:

Salad Bowl made with:
1 ½ cups of Spinach
½ Tomato
1 Carrot
2 ounces cooked and shredded lean Chicken
A handful of Walnuts
1 tablespoon of Olive Oil
1 teaspoon of Balsamic Vinegar

Snack 2:

1 cup of Popcorn
1 ounce Dark Chocolate

Dinner:

4 ounces grilled Salmon
½ cup grilled Brussel Sprouts
1/3 cup cooked Quinoa

2 Asparagus Spears
½ cup Green Grapes

Day 2:

3 Egg Whites, scrambled and cooked
4 Cherry Tomatoes
½ Avocado
A handful of Pumpkin and Sunflower Seeds (mixed)
1 glass of freshly squeezed Orange Juice

Snack 1:

1 Whole Grain Sugar-Free Plain Muffin
1 tablespoon of Peanut Butter

Lunch:

1 cup of Red Lentil Soup
1 cup of Mixed Greens drizzled with Olive Oil
1 tablespoon of Whole Grain Croutons
½ Apple

Snack 2:

1 cup Veggie Sticks (Celery, Carrots, Bell Peppers, and Zucchini)
2 tablespoons of Hummus
1 glass of fresh Lemonade (without sugar)

Dinner:

½ cup of Whole Grain Pasta
4 ounces grilled Turkey Breast
½ cup of sliced and grilled Shitake Mushrooms
½ cup Mango Chunks

Day 3:

Breakfast:

1 Smoothie made with:
- ½ Banana
- ½ Avocado
- 1 cup of Baby Spinach
- 1 tablespoon of Chia Seeds
- 1 tablespoon of Flaxseeds
- 4 Almonds
- ½ cup of Soy Milk

Snack:

1 cup of homemade Sweet Potato Chips (baked slices)
1 small Orange

Lunch:

1 whole-grain Pita Bread
1 tablespoon of Hummus
1 cup of sliced Veggies
A handful of Raisins

Snack 2:

A handful of Strawberries dipped in melted Dark Chocolate
A tablespoon of Peanuts

Dinner:

1 cup of cooked dry Kidney Beans
¼ cup of homemade Tomato Sauce (fresh tomatoes, basil, garlic, and olive oil)

1 cup of Arugula and Lettuce drizzles with Olive Oil
A handful of Red Grapes

Day 4:

Breakfast:

1 cup cooked Quinoa
¼ cup Soy Milk
1 tablespoon of Chia Seeds
¼ cup Blueberries

Snack 2:

2/3 cup of Roasted Chickpeas
1 Tangerine

Lunch:

1 cup of clear and lean Chicken Soup (made with skinless and boneless meat)
1 slices of toasted whole grain Bread
1 cup of Spinach and Cherry Tomato Salad drizzled with Olive Oil

Snack 2:

1 Apple
1 tablespoon of Almond Butter

Dinner:

4 ounces of grilled Mackerel
1/3 cup of cooked Millet
1 cup of mixed Veggies
1 ½ tablespoons of Olive Oil
A handful of Blackberries

DAY 5:

Breakfast:

3 Egg Whites, scrambled and cooked
1 slice of Whole Grain Bread, toasted
½ Avocado mashed with 1 tablespoon of Olive Oil
1 glass of freshly squeezed Orange Juice

Snack 1:

2 sugar-free Oat and Dark Chocolate Cookies
½ cup Soy Milk

Lunch:

1 cup of Creamy Veggie Soup (blended)
1 tablespoon of Pumpkin Seeds
1 tablespoon of Sunflower Seeds
1 tablespoon of Olive Oil
1 Banana

Snack 2:

A handful of Hazelnuts
4 Strawberries

Dinner:

4 ounces of lean Beef Round Steak, grilled
½ cup of mashed Potatoes and Peas drizzled with Olive Oil
4 Cherry Tomatoes
1 Peach, optional

DAY 6:

Breakfast:

1 Whole Grain English Muffin
1 tablespoon of Peanut Butter
½ cup of Soy or Almond Milk
½ Banana

Snack 1:

A handful of dried Fruit
1 tablespoon of Chia Seeds
1 cup of nonfat Greek Yogurt

Lunch:

½ cup of steamed Broccoli Florets
½ cup of cooked Brown Rice
½ cup of grilled Mushroom Slices
1/3 cup of grilled Tofu Cubes
1 tablespoon of Olive Oil
1 Apple

Snack 2:

1 Peach
A handful of Pistachios

Dinner:

1 cup of Beef Stew made with lean Beef and allowed ingredients only
1 slice of whole grain Bread
1 cup of mixed Greens drizzled with Olive Oil and Balsamic Vinegar

Day 7:

Breakfast:

1 Hardboiled Egg
½ Avocado mashed with 1 tablespoon of Olive Oil
1 Whole Grain Bread Slice, toasted
5 Olives
5 Cherry Tomatoes
1 Orange

Snack 1:

1 cup Popcorn
1 ounce Dark Chocolate

Lunch:

1 cup of Fish Soup, made with allowed ingredients
1 cup of Baby Spinach
½ cup of chopped Kale
1 ½ tablespoons of Olive Oil
1 tablespoon Pine Nuts
½ cup Grapes

Snack 2:

1 Smoothie made with:
- 1 Peach
- 4 Almonds
- ½ Banana
- 1 tablespoon Almond Butter
- 1 tablespoon Flaxseed
- 1/3 cup of Soy Milk

Dinner:

Stir fry made with:
- 2 tablespoons Olive Oil
- 4 ounces Chicken Breasts
- 1/3 cup of Bok Choy
- 1/3 cup of Broccoli
- 2 Button Mushrooms

Day 8:

Breakfast:

1 ounce Smoked Salmon
1 Whole Grain Bagel
1 Egg White, scrambled and cooked
4 Cherry Tomatoes
½ Grapefruit

Snack 1:

1 Handful of Mixed Berries
1 ounce Dark Chocolate

Lunch:

1 cup of Potato and Spinach Creamy Soup (made with allowed ingredients only)
2 tablespoons of Pine Nuts
1 Apple

Snack 2:

1 Whole Grain and Sugar-Free Cookie
½ Handful of Raisins

Dinner:

1 cup of cooked Zoodles (Zucchini Noodles)
¼ cup Homemade Tomato Sauce
3 ounces grilled Chicken
1 ounce nonfat Mozzarella Cheese
4 Olives

Day 9:

Breakfast:

1 cup of Oatmeal made with Almond Milk
2 Tangerine
2 tablespoons of Blueberries
1 ounce Dark Chocolate

Snack:

1 cup of Zucchini Chips
2 tablespoons of Cashews

Lunch:

4 grilled Scallops
½ cup Arugula
1 cup Baby Spinach
3 tablespoons of canned Chickpeas
3 Cherry Tomatoes
2 tablespoons of Olive Oil
1 Peach

Snack 2:

1 cup of Melon Chunks
A handful of Sunflower Seeds

Dinner:

½ cup cooked and shredded Turkey Meat
1 cup cooked Whole Wheat Pasta
1 tablespoon chopped Basil
2 tablespoons of Olive Oil
2 tablespoons sauted Shallots

Day 10:

Breakfast:

1 Plain English Muffin (Whole grain and sugar-free)
1 tablespoon of Peanut Butter
A handful of Raspberries
½ cup of Soy Milk

Snack 1:

½ cup nonfat Yogurt
1 tablespoon of Flaxseed
1 tablespoon of ground Almonds
½ cup Papaya Chunks

Lunch:

1 small Whole Wheat Pizza Crust
2 tablespoons homemade Tomato Sauce
A handful of Basil
1 ½ ounces Goat Cheese
3 Anchovies, chopped

Snack 2:

1 cup Popcorn
1 glass of Lemonade

Dinner:

4 ounces of lean Beef Steak, grilled
1/3 cup of cooked Wild Rice
4 Asparagus Spears, steamed
½ Tomato
½ cup Red Grapes

Day 11:

Breakfast:

½ cup of Whole Grain Granola Mix
2 tablespoons of dried Fruit
1 tablespoon of chopped Hazelnuts
2/3 cup Soy Milk

Snack 1:

½ cup of Veggie Juice
4 Whole Wheat Crackers

Lunch:

2 Bruschetta Slices made with:
- diced Tomatoes
- Basil
- Olive Oil
- No more than 1 ½ ounces of nonfat Mozzarella Cheese
1 Orange

Snack 2:

2 tablespoons of Hummus
4 Carrot Sticks
4 Celery Sticks
4 Cucumber Sticks

Dinner:

4 ounces of Rainbow Trout, grilled
½ cup baked Sweet Potato Cubes
1 cup of mixed Greens drizzled with Olive Oil

Day 12:

Breakfast:

2 Hardboiled Eggs, whites only
1 slices of Whole Wheat Bread, toasted
2 tablespoons of mashed Fruit
1 glass of Fresh Orange Juice

Snack 1:

2/3 cup Roasted Chickpeas with Turmeric Powder
1 small Fruit

Lunch:

½ cup Baby Spinach
½ cup chopped Kale
½ cup torn Lettuce
1 canned Tuna in water, drained
2 tablespoons, canned Peas
4 Cherry Tomatoes
2 tablespoons of Olive Oil
½ tablespoon of Balsamic Vinegar

Snack 2:

2 Whole Wheat and Sugar-Free Cookies (made with allowed ingredients only)
½ Apple

Dinner:

1 cup of Whole Wheat Pasta, cooked
½ cup sauted Veggies

¼ cup homemade Tomato Sauce
A Handful of Blackberries

Day 13:

Breakfast:

½ Banana
½ cup Oatmeal made with Soy Milk
1 tablespoon chopped Almonds
½ Grapefruit

Snack 1:

1 cup of chopped mixed Fruit
½ cup of nonfat Yogurt

Lunch:

1 cup of Clear Veggie Soup
1 slice of Whole Wheat Bread, TOASTED
½ Avocado mashed and drizzled with Olive Oil

Snack 2:

2 Whole Grain and Sugar-Free Biscuits (made with allowed
ingredients only: no yolks, butter, etc.)
5 Strawberries

Dinner:

½ cup cooked Barley
½ cup cooked and shredded Chicken
½ cup Salad by choice, drizzled with Olive Oil

Day 14:

Breakfast:

1 Fruity Smoothie made with:
- 1 Banana
- A handful of Strawberries
- 2 tablespoons of chopped Nuts
- 2 tablespoons of Chia Seeds
- ½ cup Soy Milk
- ¼ cup Mango Chunks

Snack 1:

1 cup of Apple Chips sprinkled with Cinnamon
A handful of Pumpkin Seeds

Lunch:

1 cup of creamy Carrot and Ginger Soup (made with allowed ingredients only)
2 tablespoons of Whole Wheat Croutons
1 tablespoon of Sunflower Seeds
1 cup of Salad by choice, with Olive Oil

Snack 2:

½ cup Papaya Chunks
1 small Whole-Wheat and Sugar-Free Granola Bar

Dinner:

4 ounces of Grilled Salmon crusted with ¼ cups Pistachios
½ cup mashed Potatoes
1/3 cup steamed Broccoli Florets
5 Strawberries dipped in melted Dark Chocolate

Day 15:

Breakfast:

1 Hardboiled Egg
1 Slice of Whole Wheat Bread, toasted
2 tbsp mashed Avocado drizzled with Olive Oil
1 Orange

Snack 1:

4 grilled Shrimp or Scallops
1 cup Veggie Juice

Lunch:

1 cup Lentil Soup
½ cup Spinach
4 Cherry Tomatoes
½ cup Arugula
A handful of Basil
3 tbsp grated Beets
2 tbsp Olive Oil

Snack 2:

½ cup nonfat Yogurt
1 tbsp Flaxseeds
2 tbsp Blueberries
1 tbsp chopped Almonds

Dinner:

1/4 cup grilled Tofu
½ cup roasted Broccoli Florets
½ Bell Pepper, roasted

¼ Onion
1 Garlic Clove
3 ounces cubed grilled Chicken
1 Peach

Day 16:

Breakfast:

1 cup cooked Quinoa
A handful of Berries
1 tbsp Flaxseeds
1 ounce Dark Chocolate
½ cup Soy Milk

Snack 1:

A handful of Raisins
4-6 Almonds

Lunch:

1 cup Baby Spinach
1 cup Lettuce
2 tbsp canned Corn
½ Tomato
¼ Cucumber
1 can Sardines in water, drained
2 tbsp Olive Oil
1 tbsp Parmesan Shavings

Snack 2:

1 Banana
1 tablespoon Almond Butter

Dinner:

Burger made with:

½ Whole Wheat Hamburger Bun
1 tbsp Dijon Mustard

4 ounces Beef pattie, grilled
¼ cup Veggie Slices
½ cup Pineapple Chunks

Day 17:

Breakfast:

2 Pancakes made with almond flour, egg whites, soy milk, and no sugar
2 tbsp mashed Fruit
½ cup nonfat Yogurt
½ Grapefruit

Snack 1:

1 cup Pretzels
1 Mango

Lunch:

½ Eggplant grilled and stuffed with:
½ cup cooked Amaranth
2 ounces cooked and shredded Chicken
½ cup sated Veggies
A handful of Greens drizzles with Olive Oil

Snack 2:

2 Homemade Cranberry and Oat Bars (made with allowed ingredients only)

Dinner:

1 cup Bean and ground Turkey Chili
½ cup Kimchi
1/2 cup Passionfruit

Day 18:

Breakfast:

1 Whole Wheat Bread Slice, toasted
1 tbsp Peanut Butter
½ Banana, sliced
½ cup Soy or Almond Milk
1 Apple

Snack 1:

1 grilled Corn on the cob sprinkled with Turmeric
1 glass of Fresh Orange Juice

Lunch:

2/3 cup cooked Orzo
2 sundried Tomatoes, chopped
2 tbsp chopped basil
1 tbsp chopped Parsley
3 ounces cooked and shredded Chicken
1 ounce nonfat Mozzarella Cheese

Snack 2:

A handful of Pistachios
1 Apricot

Dinner:

4 ounces Mackerel
½ cup mashed Sweet Potato with Turmeric

Day 19:

Breakfast:

1 cup cooked Oats
½ cup Soy Milk
½ cup chopped mixed Fruit
1 tbsp chopped Hazelnuts
1 Tangerine

Snack 1:

2/3 cup baked Tortilla Chops
½ cup Guacamole
1 glass of Lemonade

Lunch:

1 cup of clean Chicken Soup
½ whole wheat Pita Bread
½ cup chopped Papaya

Snack 2:

1 cup Sweet Potato cubes with Turmeric
1 glass of Blackberry Juice (homemade and sugar-free)

Dinner:

1 cup cooked whole wheat Penne
¼ cup homemade Pesto Sauce (with allowed ingredients)
1/3 cup cooked and shredded Turkey
½ cup Grapes

Day 20:

Breakfast:

Omelet made with:
- 1 Egg
- 2 Egg Whites
- 1/3 cup sliced Green Onions
- 1/3 cup sliced Mushrooms
- 4 Cherry Tomatoes
- ½ Whole Wheat Toast

Snack 1:

1 cup Popcorn
1 ounce Dark Chocolate

Lunch:

1 cup Green Mix
1 Tomato, chopped
1 can Tuna in water, drained
2 tbsp Corn
¼ cup ground Almonds

Snack 2:

1 Whole-Whet Plain Muffin
1 tbsp mashed Fruit

Dinner:

1 Veggie Pattie, grilled
½ cup mashed Cauliflower
4 steamed Asparagus Spears

½ cup Red Cabbage drizzled with Olive Oil
1 Nectarine

Day 21:

Breakfast:

1 cup of Oatmeal cooked with Soy Milk
1 tbsp Applesauce
1 tbsp Blueberries
1 tbsp Chiaseeds
1 tbsp chopped Nuts
½ Grapefruit

Snack 1:

1 Banana
4 Pecans

Lunch:

1 cup Cauliflower Rice (ground in food processor)
2 tbsp canned diced Tomatoes
½ cup chopped roasted Veggies
1 ounce nonfat Mozzarella Cheese
½ Apple

Snack 2:

4 Baby Carrots
2 tbsp Hummus
4 Celery Sticks
1 Tangerine

Dinner:

4 ounces grilled Salmon
½ cup cooked Quinoa

½ cup Veggies
2 tbsp dried Fruit

Conclusion

See? Following a triglyceride-lowering diet is not as overwhelming as you thought. The food combinations are pretty much endless, and with this book's meal plan you can never run out of cooking ideas.

Now that you know what you need to do, the next step is to bring your triglyceride levels within the normal range. Once you do that, you can then go full Mediterranean and pack your kitchen with the amazing flavors of Greece and Italy.

You can help me and your fellow readers by leaving a review on Amazon and sharing your thoughts on this book. You have no idea how much this would help!

One last thing. How would you like winning a **$200.00 Amazon Gift Card** and helping me improve this book in the process with a little bit of feedback?

That's right :)

Your opinion is so valuable to me that I am giving away a $200 gift card to *the luckiest one of 200 participants*!

It will only take a minute of your time to let me know what you like and what you didn't like about this book. The hardest part is deciding how to spend the two hundred dollars!

Just follow this link.

http://booksfor.review/triglycerides

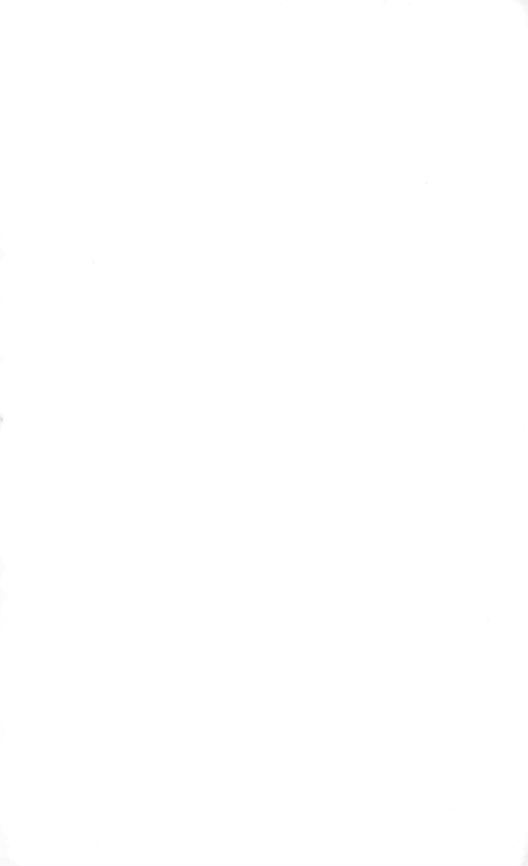

Printed in Great Britain
by Amazon

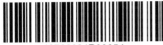

48722684R00054